Illustrated Hints for Health and Strength for Busy People;

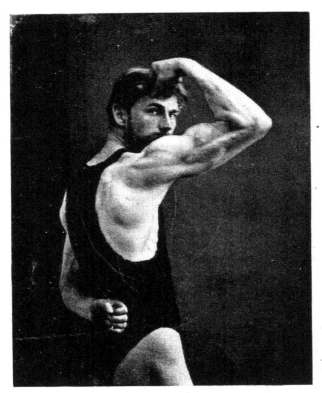

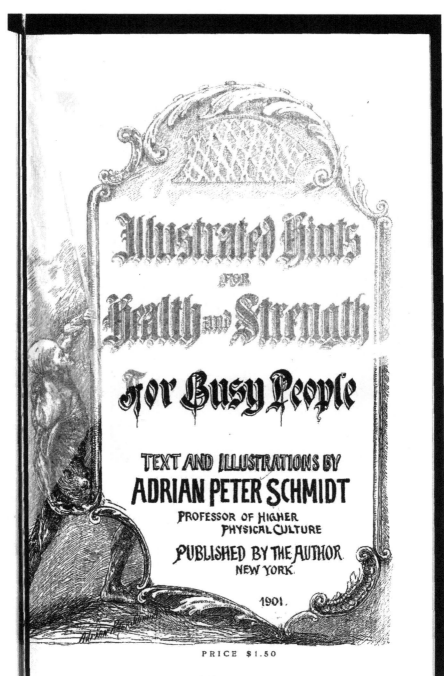

Illustrated Hints

for

Health and Strength

for Busy People

TEXT AND ILLUSTRATIONS BY

ADRIAN PETER SCHMIDT

PROFESSOR OF HIGHER
PHYSICAL CULTURE

PUBLISHED BY THE AUTHOR.
NEW YORK.

1901.

PRICE $1.50

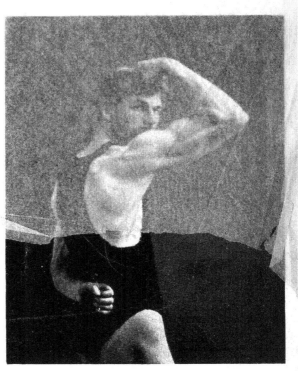

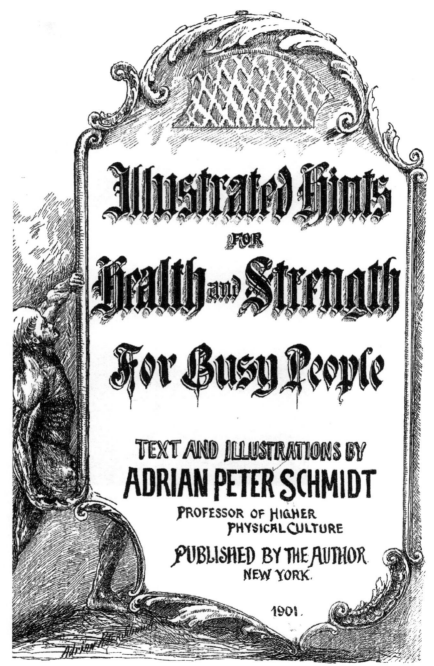

Illustrated Hints
for
Health and Strength
For Busy People

TEXT AND ILLUSTRATIONS BY

ADRIAN PETER SCHMIDT

PROFESSOR OF HIGHER
PHYSICAL CULTURE

PUBLISHED BY THE AUTHOR
NEW YORK.

1901.

Copyright, 1901
By Adrian Peter Schmidt

Redfield Brothers, New York

PREFATORY NOTE

The subject of this book has been treated concisely to save the reader's time

Anticipating the difficulty of following, successfully, instructions generally given in books, the author has spent considerable time and care upon the pen and ink drawings illustrating his instructions.

The exercises described herein have been carefully tested from a strictly physiological point of view. They can safely be practiced by persons of middle age or beyond, contrary to an existing popular impression that active physical exercise should be avoided at that stage of life.

The author's aim has been, not to write upon an interesting subject for mere casual reading, but to present a practical manual for continuous use.

E N D O R S E M E N T S

The manual should be of very great value to all persons who are in search of a short road to sound health and thorough physical development, embodying as it does, an intelligible and concise presentation of the excellent methods of rational physical culture, taught by the author in his institute, and by which all who have studied under him have profited.

We, who have enjoyed the opportunity of testing the methods and theories of Professor Adrian Peter Schmidt, take great pleasure in sincerely and heartily recommending this manual to all who are interested in this subject.

CLARENCE H. MACKAY
New York

G. BAUMANN
Holland House, New York — Chicago

(REV. DR.) CHAS. H. BABCOCK
New York

JAMES D. W. CUTTING
Knickerbocker Club, N. Y.

CARL BERGER
New York — Newport, R. L.

JAMES H. BEEKMAN
Union Club, N. Y.

DANIAL A. DAVIS
New York

E. W. COGGESHALL
New York

DAVID B. OGDEN
New York

FRANK S. THOMAS
New York Athletic Club

GEO. HERRMANN
New York

J. O. LOWSON JOHNSTON
New York — London

CHAS. J. McBURNEY
New York

COUNT ALEXANDER HADECK
Abroad

INDEX OF ILLUSTRATIONS

A FEW SUGGESTIONS
as to PHYSICAL CULTURE
FOR BUSY PEOPLE

E are living in times that demand more and more of our brains and muscles, of our nerves and physical energy. Only those who are strong, and know how to keep so, can stand the wear and tear.

It pays to stop once in a while to look over our machinery and oil the parts that need it. Failing to do this we will find our capacity for work growing less, until at last we will be compelled to stop, giving to others the place that we might have filled for many years longer with benefit to ourselves and others.

A due proportion of exercise is essential to the perfect working of the functions of the physical and mental man. Good judgment, quick thought, self control and will power—so necessary in these busy days—cannot be retained for any length of time by anyone who does not pay proper attention to his physical condition; deplorable results will follow, either because of erroneous notions or sheer carelessness.

Proper exercise causes the blood to circulate throughout the entire body nourishing all its parts; from the lack of exercise the body is unable to maintain its vigor, and the mind, whose health is dependent upon that of the body, is soon reduced to a condition of languor.

So many have written on the importance of physical exercise, that it would be unprofitable to reiterate statements that everybody has read over and over again and the truth of which all are willing to concede.

My purpose is a very practical one—to suggest a simple plan for exercise in the morning, which will take only ten or fifteen minutes, but whose practical and beneficial results have been demonstrated in my experience as an advisor and instructor in physical culture.

The exercises do not require any apparatus and can be taken in a room large enough for you to turn around in with outstretched arms. Of course good ventilation is essential.

If you practice these exercises intelligently and persistently they will put you in a condition to go through your daily work with ease and pleasure.

2

Violent exercise (by this I do not mean vigorous exercise) should be avoided early in the morning, as the condition of the body is rather languid just after awakening from a night's sleep, and would produce too sudden a change in the circulation of the blood. A cold bath without previous exercise should be avoided for the same reason, the stimulation being too severe and the reaction, though sometimes pleasant, is anything but invigorating, as depression soon follows.

Be moderate in the beginning.

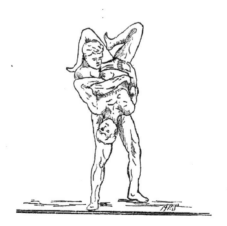

3

𝕻late I

Here is a simple and rather ingenious plan to stimulate energy in a mild way on mornings when you do not feel inclined to exert your strength.

Take in each hand a corner of an ordinary sheet of newspaper (any kind of soft paper will do) and crumple it up until the four corners are brought into the palms of your hands, forming paper balls. Avoid assisting in the process by pressing the hands against the body. The result is surprising. Every muscle will be brought into sympathy with the muscles of the forearm in the effort to secure the last corner (to completely hide the sheets in your hands). Your nervous force and blood circulation are thus pleasantly stimulated.

Practice this from one to two minutes, beginning slowly and gradually increasing in speed.

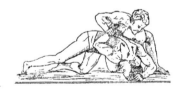

4

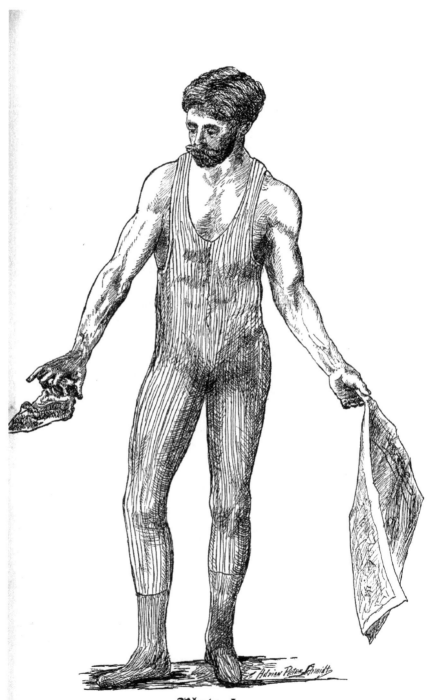

Plate I

Plate II

REMARK: Using these paper balls in the same manner as a grip-machine, by grasping them as tightly as you can and then releasing the grip without opening the fingers entirely, repeating this about seventy-five times a minute, will insure a powerful grip. Simple as this paper grip-machine seems, it is superior in many ways to any manufactured device.

The writer has carried one in his coat pocket in cold weather to keep his hands warm by exercise and has repeatedly illustrated the strength of his fingers by tearing a corner off a full deck of cards, lifting with one finger a good-sized man by the belt, etc., feats that anyone can perform after persistent exercise.

This exercise does not make the hands callous nor enlarge or deform the joints. It massages the flesh covering the inside of the hands, including the thumb, and gives them beautiful outlines.

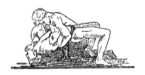

6

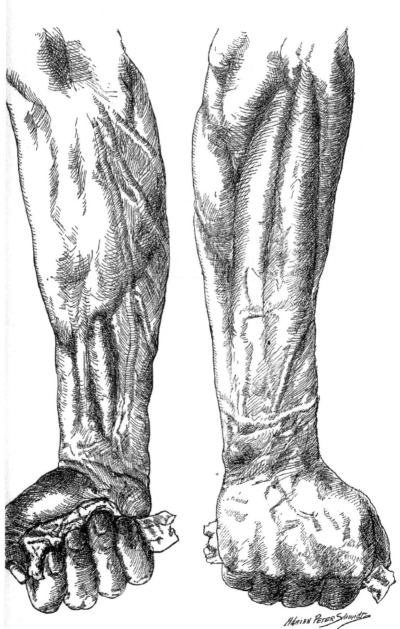

ADRIAN PETER SCHMIDT

𝔓late III

Very effective exercise for the muscles of the neck, the upper trapezius muscles that cover most of the upper part of the back and deltoids or ᐟ shoulder muscles.

Stand erect in a comfortable, natural position, bringing the outstretched arms sideways, with fists clinched, knuckles upward, elbows straight on a horizontal line with the shoulders. Compare your position in a mirror with illustration. (You can use paper balls for the convenience of having something to steady your fingers.)

Rotate arms, making fists travel in circles of about seven to ten inches in diameter, spending most of the energy on half circle marked with X on the dotted line.

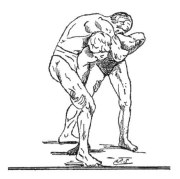

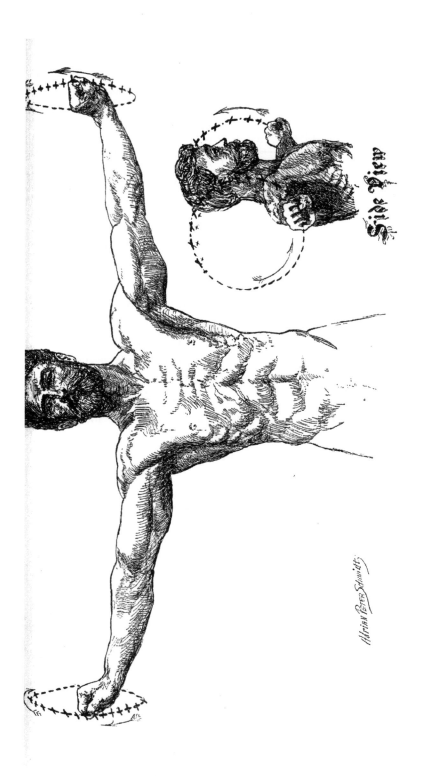

Side View

Plate IV

Arms the same as in Plate III, trunk inclined forward, knuckles downward. For convenience bring one leg forward, bending the knee as much as is comfortable. Reverse the rotation of your arms.

This exercise developes that part of the shoulder muscles, the absence of which your tailor supplies by padding your coat.

Begin the rotations slowly, laying stress on reaching as far sideways as possible, then gradually increase the speed. Continue the rotations for one minute in each position (III and IV) from forty to one hundred times, according to your strength. After this exercise the shoulders will require a rest.

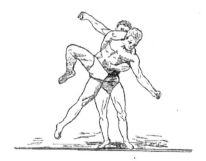

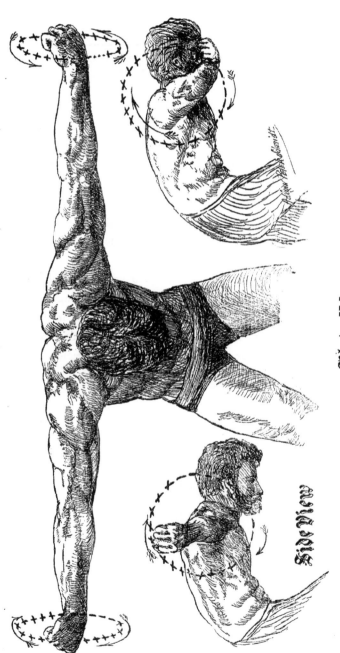

Side View

Plate IV

Plate V

To stimulate the circulation in the lower extremities and develop the strength of their muscles.

Standing erect and without bending at the hips, raise heels and toes alternately from thirty to sixty times according to your strength and the time at your disposal. One minute will be sufficient

Illustrations A, B, C and D show the various feet positions in which this exercise may be taken so as to bring into play the different calf muscles. It is advisable to take from eight to fifteen exercises in each position

This exercise should be taken barefooted or in stockings on a soft rug. Raise as high as you can, avoiding dropping the heels suddenly.

If you have difficulty in keeping your balance, steady yourself by holding on to the back of a chair or to a door-knob.

REMARK: Avoid going to extremes at first, as the calf muscles are liable to become painfully sore the next day.

12

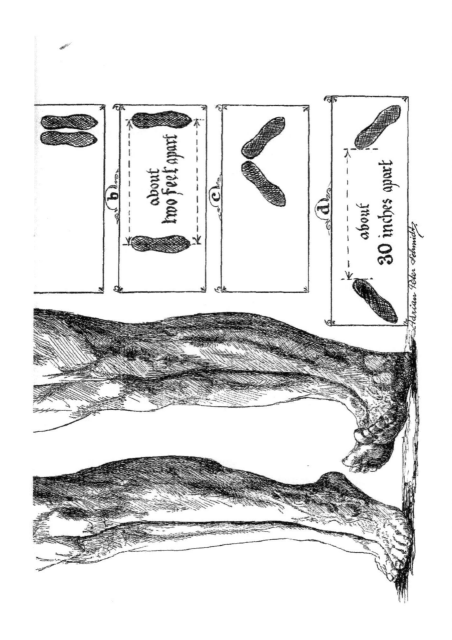

b.

about
two feet apart

c.

d.

about
30 inches apart

Adrian Peter Schmidt

Plate VI

After previous exercise with the weight of your body alternately on the heels and toes, the accumulation of venous blood gives rise to a tired sensation in the leg muscles.   To remove this temporary congestion immediately, lift the right foot off the floor, bending the knee, supporting the weight of the limb as shown in illustration IV   Move feet from ankles a few turns to the right and a few to the left; then up and down   Do the same with the left foot. If your time is limited operate both feet at the same time, sitting on a chair, bed or lounge.

An elaborate explanation of the physiological effects of this exercise would take too much space and be of little service to the busy reader.

I can earnestly recommend it for cold feet, stiff ankles and toe joints, headaches resulting from various causes, catarrhal inflammation of the mucous membrane of the nostrils, etc.   Provided you don't wear tight shoes this exercise V and VI can be practiced at any time with good results.

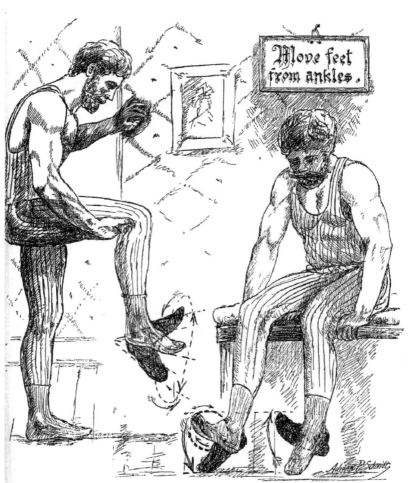

Plate VI

𝕻late VII

To cleanse the lungs of all impurities that may have accumulated during the night and increase the blood circulation :

Take two or three deep breaths, entirely emptying lungs, and then filling them to their fullest capacity. Standing erect, reach upward keeping elbows and knees straight, fists clinched or fingers outstretched as you please, and feet comfortably apart, say about the width of your shoulders. Bring the body from position A to position B repeatedly in a rather slow rhythm.

Lift chin up when in erect position A (avoid leaning backward), inhale slowly through the nose until the lungs are completely filled, elevate the shoulders as high as you can and draw the abdominal walls inward : then release abdominal walls and bring the body into position B exhaling through the nose or mouth as you please, bending the knees, bringing the armpits close to the knees or touching them if you are able to do so, attempting to touch the floor with the hands about sixteen or eighteen inches from the feet

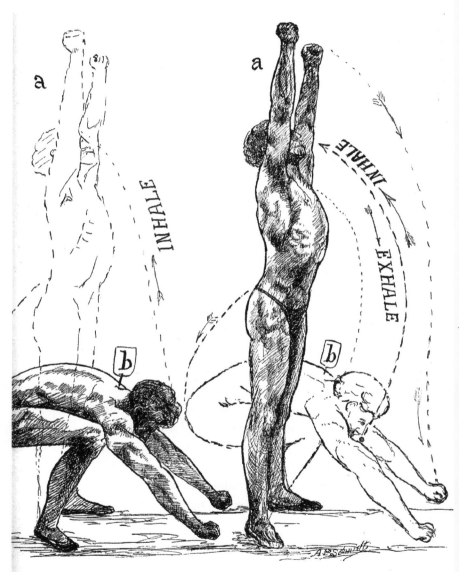

REPEAT ABOUT FIFTEEN TIMES WHICH WILL
REQUIRE ABOUT ONE MINUTE

Plate VII

Plate VIII

To stimulate circulation in the abdominal cavity and invigorate the muscles surrounding and enfolding the assimilative and vital organs, which by reflex action of the muscles are themselves invigorated.

This exercise is practiced lying on the floor on some soft yielding but firm surface. A rug folded lengthwise or a bed-comfortable will do. An excellent exercise-mat may be made from inch or two inch pipe-felting, covered with canvas in size three by six or eight feet.

Bring the body from position A to B (or IX–C as you are able) by throwing your outstretched arms with an energetic semi-circular forward motion towards your feet or knees, following with the head and shoulders

Avoid holding your breath while going from position A to B but expel the air from your lungs by exclaiming "whoo", this assists, as it brings the abdominal muscles into play.

Avoid relaxing the muscles suddenly when going back into position A as the jar resulting is unpleasant and not beneficial.

18

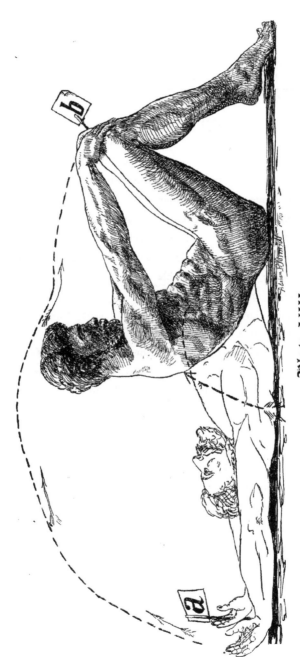

Plate VIII

𝕻late IX

It may be found difficult to follow these instructions strictly at first because of a certain amount of stiffness in the knees, hips, spine and shoulder joints, or weakness in the abdominal muscles, which are to be looked for in people of sedentary habits.

But no matter how little progress you make at first, steadily persist in your efforts to overcome these conditions and you will be amply rewarded.

Stout men will lose a great deal of superfluous fat around the waist line in attempting this exercise, as the increase of strength of the abdominal muscles destroys all fatty tissues which hamper their action.

If you are not able to reach to your knees without lifting the feet from the ground, lift them or reach only to the thighs, but try to do better next time.

The gradual development of the abdominal muscles insures a safeguard against ruptures.

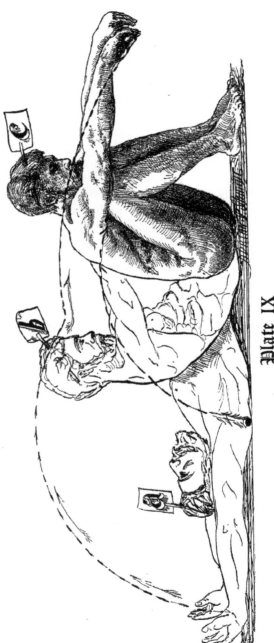

Plate XI

Dumb bells, of from one to five pounds in weight, will assist you on account of the increased momentum they will give.

The number of consecutive exercises of this kind must depend upon the condition and good judgment of the reader. Should your limit be five, then rest a few seconds and take five more and so on until you have taken twenty-five or exercised in this way for at least two or three minutes.

I would impress upon my reader the great importance of this kind of exercise to health.

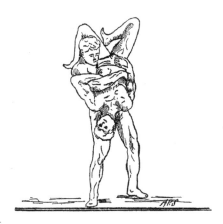

22

The alternate practice of exercise (Plate VIII or IX) and the following exercise (Plate X) has proven to be of great assistance for the elimination of gases produced by fermentation of food.

This imperfect digestion is generally produced by: large quantities of fluids taken with meals, especially ice water; food taken while in a state of nervousness; prolonged mental overwork; hasty eating; deficient mastication; late suppers, followed by insufficient sleep; insomnia and numerous complications.

The digestive functions and the nervous system act and react reciprocally.

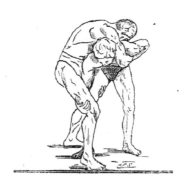

𝔓late X

As the reverse of exercise VIII or IX in which the abdominal muscles are chiefly involved and the spine strongly and repeatedly brought into a convex curve, take the following exercise for the back muscles and spine.

Lie on your abdomen with the legs in a comfortable position, chin (or forehead) resting on the folded arms.

Consecutively raise elbows, head and chest together (the chin or forehead not leaving the arms during the exercise) from two to nine inches, according to your ability, from A to B as shown in illustration, with a spring-like motion, not stopping at A. Avoid striking the floor with the elbows—put the energy in the rising motion. The lumbar region is thus vigorously brought into action.

REMARK : Practice this exercise with forehead resting on arms, if not able to occupy illustrated position, until joints in neck gain suppleness.

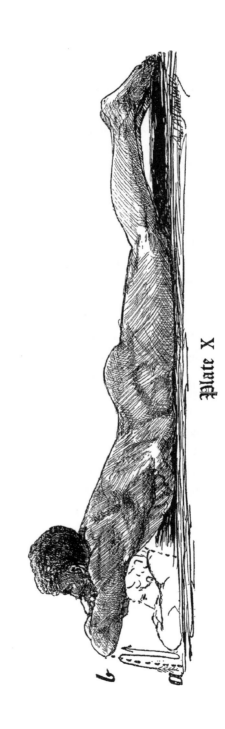

Plate X

Persons past middle age will probably have some difficulty in raising higher than an inch or two at first and will feel exhausted after five or six consecutive attempts. They should rest a few seconds after four or five exercises, but increase the height of the rise and the number of times in proportion with their gain of muscular strength and suppleness of spine. One minute will be sufficient.

Few minutes spent daily in this exercise will soon result in correcting the round backs which are caused by sitting with in-sunken chest, by exaggerated bicycle riding, etc.

I have given this exercise with surprising results, even to men of sixty years of age.

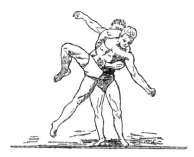

26

Persons troubled with constipation, which is often produced by sedentary habits, will find the practice of exercises VIII or IX, X and XI, alternately, an effective remedy.

Quite a number of other exercises, combined with rational diet, will be found beneficial in such cases, varying as they do as to the causes and the constitution, but it would be outside of the writer's present purpose to treat of them exhaustively here.

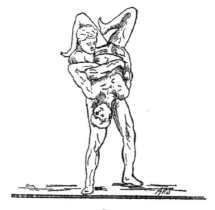

𝔓late XI

This exercise is rather difficult to illustrate, but simple in execution.

It is like a rocking chair in motion, the spine being the rocker. The body is doubled up as shown in illustration and this attitude is kept throughout the massage exercise.

Start this exercise by sitting down, clasping the hands below the knees, roll into position B and, without stopping there, roll back into the sitting position without unclasping your hands or changing the convex curve of your spine—in other words, throw your body from the sitting position A into shoulder position B and back into A with an uninterrupted rolling motion, occupying about three seconds. Repeat two or three minutes, taking an occasional rest so that your breathing may become normal.

Don't hold your breath, but breathe as naturally as possible.

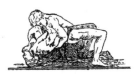

28

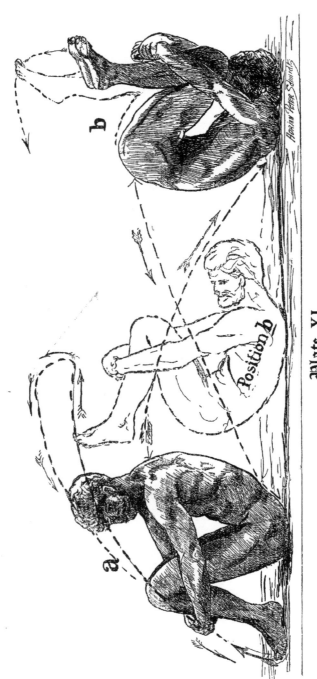

Position b

b

a

Plate XI

Plate XII

That the tonic effect of a cold bath upon the nervous system may be fully obtained, it should always be preceded by sufficient exercise to put the body in a glow—but do not take your bath until you breathe naturally and the heart has resumed its normal action.

It should be taken in such a manner as to wet the body all over, beginning with the head, then shoulders, chest, back and limbs, requiring in all only from two to six seconds.

Before rubbing yourself, cover every part of your body with a bath robe or bath sheet made of Turkish towelling, which is preferable to any other material because it will absorb the water rapidly. (If you have no such robe or sheet get into bed.)

Do not fail to cover your feet also, that they may feel the general reaction which follows immediately upon covering yourself with the bath robe. Rub your hair well with a towel until dry (it strengthens the roots of the hair) and then after the reaction has fully taken place rub any part of the body that feels wet and follow this by a general friction with your hands or a towel, beginning with the limbs and following with the trunk, shoulders and arms.

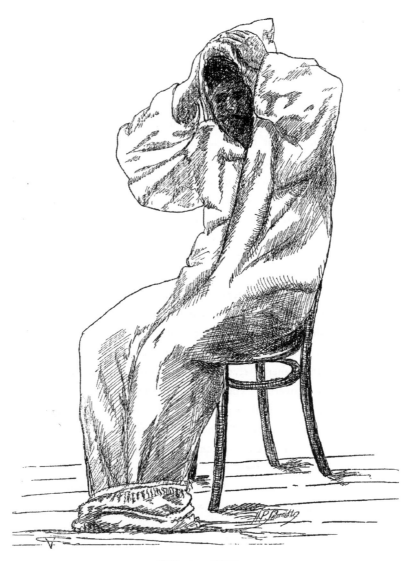

Plate XII

I wish to emphasize the benefit derived from thoroughly wrapping up the body after the cold water application. It hastens the reaction and makes it uniform, as it checks the loss of heat all over the body at the same time. This is of special importance to people who are not in vigorous health.

Those who think that cold water baths do not agree with them will probably change their opinion after a trial of this method.

The writer hopes that he has redeemed his promise of a few simple suggestions and that their value will be appreciated by all who make use of them.

ADRIAN PETER SCHMIDT
167 West 57th Street, New York
Opposite Carnegie Music Hall

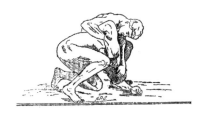

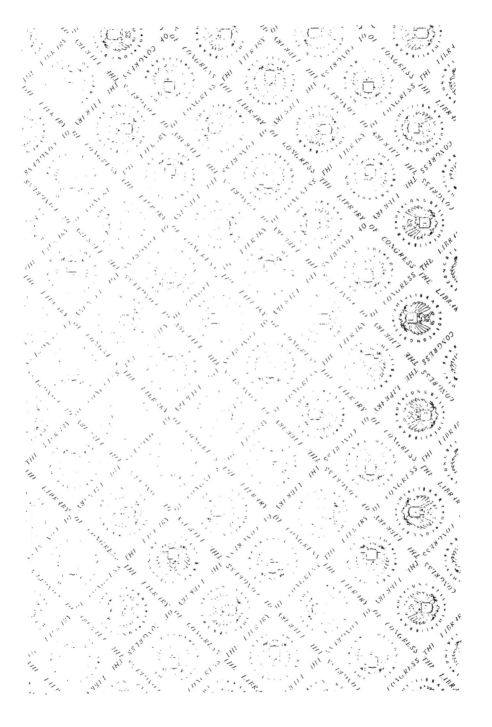

Ingram Content Group UK Ltd.
Milton Keynes UK
UKHW020119200523
422059UK00005B/62

9 781015 523852